HONEY-BASED RECIPES

For Beginners

Taylah Greenway

Contents

Chapter One

THE BOOK

INTRODUCTION

You can skip this section if you are not interested in the menu.

My mother wrote this cookbook for my sister and I when we were kids and we grew up on the Blueberry Hill series of cookbooks written by her (I'm a triplet). Blueberry Hill books, including this one, grew out of the recipe-sharing tradition in Mary Jane's Kitchen, which I wrote about in this chapter. I've changed some of the recipes to accommodate our preferences, including less fat and less sugar, and I have tried to include my top restaurants to satisfy us grown-ups when we're not café eating.

And now, I will introduce each chapter around a distinctive nut. You may cook with these nuts, but I also have alternative suggestions in case you do not have all of the nuts I am suggesting. I have listed the alternative nuts in the back of the book.

As he describes a beekeeper's work in each season, Miller draws parallels to his own experiences in the mountains of western North Carolina. He also discusses the affect of pollen on bee health and provides examples of the work that takes up much of a beekeeper's time. This book is for bee garden enthusiasts and backyard or small-scale beekeepers.

Choose recipes that you can adapt to your tastes. If you live close to where you can get the freshest produce possible, you will improve the connection between you and your food.

Honey has a sweet taste and nourishes our bodies. Honey is a bioactive ingredient and the bees who pollinate it are very important in the food chain. Without bees, none of the fruits we enjoy in our food would thrive. Honey improves your health and is the perfect treat on any dessert!

I am happy to introduce you (and all my listeners) to some of my favorite honeys: a Pasadena-based honey seller, an organic honey from Colorado, and a honey from Maryland. Joey brings out wonderful, fresh, organic honey in small, delicious portions. Her husband Jay is a hobby hive keeper who is able to provide a raw honey that is less processed than most commercial honeys. Both of them share their knowledge with all my listeners. Johnny is a hard-

Bee-Dependent Ingredients

In each of the recipes, honeybees are noted in bold.

How to Eat Honey

Honey has many definitions. Some sources say it is produced by bees when bees forage on flower nectar and return to the hive to deposit honey. Others say honey is a sweet, edible substance secreted by glands producing a variable percentage of water and various carbohydrates and fats. Honey also refers to glutinous substances produced by certain mammals for the purpose of pleasure, and also may mean any liquid with a sweet, sweet, taste. Honey could be a sweet, edible liquid secreted by an animal.

I thought of this article about taste testing honey and decided to collect honey from different locations to study and taste.

The sights, smells, and tastes are broken into three parts: sight, smell, and taste.

Sight

Honey really is a magical foodstuff! You can make many different dishes and use it for a lot of different things. When it comes to the consistency of honey, I think you should know that you will not be able to tell a crystallized honey from a liquid honey. But once you know what consistency of honey you are looking at, you can identify a jar of too thin honey — a

What you are actually seeing is the presence of insects and pests in raw, unprocessed honey that is too pure to eat or be used in cooking. Most European beekeepers remove these contaminants or organisms through filtration, but if you are concerned about it, you may ask your be

What color is it? The honey can be very light or dark, from wheat to dark brown. Helping to describe the color of your honey can help others identify it.

Smell

Honey has a distinctive aroma that can easily be detected. The aroma varies from unadulterated honey to that of rotten honey. The sweet smell of honey comes from the tiny amounts of sugar dissolved in the honey. Handle it with care, and you will not have any of this sweet smell a day after purchasing honey.

The likelihood of this honey contradicting the USDA food safety database increases as the honey ownership increases; see page 11. Honey taste preferences are somewhat predetermined. However, honey sweetens the nation's palate without sugar. To use the honey flavor wheel on page 17, start in the center of the wheel and pick which of the seven descriptors most fits your perception of the taste of the honey. Does it have a floral aroma? Is it a warm, vegetal, woody, chemical, fresh, or fruity smell? Or does it smell

Inside each pie shaped entrance in the wheel, text (like *warm*, *burned*, *cooked*, and *caramelized*) that describe the smell can be read to define the smell better. The smell of *warm*

It is very important to note that everyone's senses have subtle differences and the taste of honey differs from person to person. Some love strong dark honeys while others love light, mild ones. Despite these different preferences, no two people are alike.

Taste

Take one small bite of the honey by setting it on a toothpick. You do not have to pour a whole puddle onto a plate!

There are several flavors around us. Some of us taste the difference between honey and grape juice, while others taste the difference between pine and lemon. Some of us love the sweet taste of honey, while some do not like that of salt. Some of us love the flavor of a sweet lemon, while others say the same about a bitter lime.

If someone asks you what you find in the flavor wheel, follow the second aroma descriptor around the perimeter of the wheel. If after sampling honey, you notice the term woody, follow the center of the wheel around to nutmeg. The spice in the flavor wheel is coffee.

Don't be surprised if you find out that honey tastes slightly different on every palate and there's no one way to enjoy it.

It takes a little practice to learn to taste honey, but it gets easier with a little practice. Honey tasting, I find, is fun because I am able to remember different honeys a lot more easily than other things I taste. (For more information on honey tasting, see my book, The Secrets of Honey Tasting.)

Honey flavor wheel

The center of the wheel is where the honey originates. The compounds in the honey are refined and the sweet taste is carried out.

What's Happening In the Hive?

Where I live, it is a quieter time in the hive during the winter. In the United States, the European honey bee is a domesticated bee. Therefore, they are easy to keep and are kept in homes to pollinate crops. As a domesticated bee, they are more likely to be put into a bag and "tak king down the country."

Shoveling snow during the winter from driveway to sidewalk and back again is exhausting work for carp and macaw workers. During the summer, they might work for a month, but during the winter they work for six months without a break.

As the weather becomes warmer, colonies begin to move honey as a surplus energy source to be stored for the coming summer. Weakened from winter, often the bees are more active and exhibit behavior different from previous years. Bees will be getting ready to swarm, so the beekeeper needs to be vigilant to keep an eye on the hive. During this time, it is also important to clean, inspect, and repair bee equipment.

Some beekeepers can make a quick check on the bee farms by being able to see the hives and the honey which they have stored. These beekeepers can then decide whether to add a feeder with their own honey to their bees.

There are some happenings that, if they are not wholly poetic and truth-telling, at least point towards a nobler and better way to relate to nature than we know. One good example of this would be the practice of bee-keeping.

—

Impress your friends with a featured tasting note

Orange Blossom Honey <|endoftext|>

Colors: Light yellow/orange

Smell: Mild and fresh, like flowers

Has a: Bitter, sour citrus flavor, and an orange rind aftertaste.

Flavor: Mild, with a short for having a lasting aftertaste

In keeping with its name, orange blossom honey is......

Meyer Lemon- and Honey-Marinated Chicken Skewers

How many servings are there in a cup? 6 as an appetizer.

If you can't find these lemons, conventional lemons will work, but Meyer lemons will give the chicken a distinctive and memorable flavor. Though it started as a purely savory recipe, I think it works very well with a bit of honey. And it's super simple. This is a perfect starter recipe for a honey themed dinner.

It's a thought: Have an appetizer party using all the appetizers in this book. Fun! (Very useful for a budget-conscious party planner.)

The ingredients

For the chicken

- 1 **Meyer lemon**
- 2 cloves of garlic crushed
- 1 teaspoon salt
- ½ teaspoon freshly ground black pepper • ½ teaspoon cayenne pepper
- Two tablespoons of extra-virgin olive oil

So, you want a tablespoon of honey, something that you probably have in your kitchen already. 2 • cinnamon •

- 15 chopsticks **white** 2 jalapeno peppers **green** 3
- Who wants to know?

A For the dipping sauce thingy.

The popular culture of Greek yogurt consists of a handful of different brands, and it's easy to grab a bowl when you're in need of a quick snack.

- Enough to coat 2 tablespoons of honey
- ZES**T** 1 **O**
- 2 cups orange juice

For the skewers

25

- ¼ pound button mushrooms
- 1/2 pound **pearl onions** (if making fresh, use this number**or** prepared pearl onions)
- **red bell pepper**, seeded and sliced in squares, 1 inch

Bold = foods that are pollinated or produced by bees

Read more here about what you can do

1.Wash the lemon and juice it (yes, this includes the rind). Put the juice into a medium bowl, add the garlic, salt, pepper, olive oil, honey, and red wine. Mix and allow it to sit on the countertop overnight. For 1 hour before cooking, add your chicken cubes and allow to marinade in the refrigerator overnight.

For the dipping sauce, combine the yogurt, honey, orange blossom honey, and orange juice in a small bowl, stirring until well mixed. Refrigerate until used. When you use a paraphrasing tool, you can search

Three. Bring the skewers to a medium-hot fire on a charcoal or gas grill. Soak the skewers in water for at least thirty minutes to keep them from burning.

Divide the mushrooms, pearl onions, bell pepper, and chicken into equal portions. Put the chicken on last.

Grill a rack of pork ribs for 3 minutes per side, flipping and re-grilling the rack after each side is cooked.

You can serve this dish with a dipping sauce.

Noticeable Characteristics

In the summer during high productivity, a worker bee lives for 42 to 45 days. In a cold winter, a worker could live for 6 months. The queen can live for 4 or 5 years. Some say she is reduced to an impotent state after two years. Derision of such a contention would involve nothing more than a discussion as to how to express

Identify the three main varieties of honey

To make honey, honeybees collect nectar that they then convert with an enzyme into high-energy sugar, one that is easy to absorb. They then put this sweet liquid into empty cells of a comb much like a corkboard, but their bee.

Worker bees dislodge any insect larvae that are inside the comb and fan the comb. The bees then clean the comb, removing any remaining insect larvae. At that point, the bees put a wax cap on the comb and wait for it to dry. When the comb is finished drying

A specific honey varietal is the result of careful observation of honey-producing plants in a place where there are no other plants. Bees will collect nectar from the plants and deposit their honey in the honeycomb, ensuring that it will be only honey of one particular variety and yield.

Many beekeepers who strive to accumulate a large number of purebred bees cannot often move their hives or harvest a wide selection of varieties. I call this honey a “stoney knob gold” because it is a reflection of the floral and other scents from my neighborhood. I taste the unique flavors of my bees as I inhale noisily from their honeycomb. Honey made by the bees of my home is truly a work of art.

Tuscan Raspberry Orange Slices with Berry Sauce

Serves 8

I adore this soup, especially when I suddenly find that customers are coming to my store. It helps me get my day started in the morning. I also make it frequently for soup suppers when my shop needs something a little different to offer customers.

The ingredients

• 4 **garlic** cloves, peeled

1 cup olive oil.

• 1 small red onion - sliced thinly

• **red bell pepper**, cut into large chunks. 2 **fettuccine pasta**, dried Paraphrase: **fettuccine pasta**,

• A **yellow bell pepper seeded and cut into 2 large chunks**

<

• Two 28-ounce cans whole tomatoes (San Marzano are great).

Navel orange is so orange that it can be cut across for wedges and then into thin circles or slices. Orange can be easily peeled away and thus does not need to be removed just before

•

• 1 cup shredded Parmesan cheese • • • 2-3 people, depending on the size of the pizza Paraphrase: • 2-3 people • depends on the size

[Bold] = foods pollinated or produced by bees

Here's what you should do

1. 1. Sauté the garlic cloves in olive oil in a medium soup pot over low heat for 3 minutes. Then add the onion and bell peppers, and continue cooking for about 5 minutes, or until the onions and bell peppers are soft.

2. 2.Add the tomatoes. I like a lot of texture in my soup, so I usually coarsely cut the tomatoes with a knife and fork once they are in the pot. Add the orange slices. Simmer for 20 minutes or so.

Some canned tomatoes are very salty and others less so. I have a salt grinder in my kitchen and season the soup with a little salt and pepper before serving. The orange slices will taste sweet.

With chunks of more vegetables and the cauli rice, this soup has a more bready taste. If you prefer a smoother texture, pour it into a food processor or blender and pulse until you have the desired texture.

4. What to do with the finished dish. Garnish with shaved Parmesan and get ready for compliments.

Papa's Salad with Clementines

Serves 8

My mother's grandfather ran a general store, where she and her apple pie baking became a star. The sugar in the original recipe was honey and it became my mother's preference when she moved to a school cafeteria job in my father's town. The citrus flavors that came through as she baked this dish in the kitchen had an influence on my interpretation of the flavors in the salad today. It's become one of my favorite dishes.

The ingredients

For the salad

• 1 head Boston lettuce (or local Bibb)

head lettuce • | | 2 | 3 wards | Tail baby romaine lettuce Paraphrase:

• • • • **cucumber**, sliced into thin rounds.

1 small nutty **onion**, sliced into thin rounds

• Shredded romaine with thinly sliced radishes

• 2 clementines, peeled and sectioned, white parts removed

• 2 hard-boiled eggs, peeled and sliced into rounds

For the dressing

• Use as much honey as you like

• 2 Tablespoons Vinegar

• ½ cup half-and-half

• Season Coarse salt and freshly ground black pepper (optional)

Bees pollinate or produce bold and colorful foods

Here's what you can do

Cut the pay bill into quarters.

Add the lettuce, cucumber, onion, radishes, clementines, and eggs (in that order) to a large decorative ceramic or wooden bowl.

Pour the honey and vinegar mixture into a medium sized bowl, whisking as you do so, and add the half-and-half.

Put about 2/3 teaspoon of Dijon mustard in the salad dressing, and toss it very gently with the salad. (This step may be omitted if the older ones eat salad dressing with their lunch.)

Before you start: Take the bowl to the table. Tell your guests: about my grandfather.

Try in the summer.

This salad is made with a variety of local ingredients that are already available to be discovered in your local farmer's market, which allows for a more authentic flavor.

Tenderloin, pork

Serves 6

Good quality pork is complemented by both sweet and hot flavors. On a visit to Italy, I was wowed by a pork dish that used local honey. After making this dish numerous times, I decided to experiment, using honey and fresh fruit. Here is what I came up with.

The ingredients

• Two pounds of pork tenderloins

They soaked two slices of bread in olive oil, on both sides. Then they put them under the broiler for about two minutes, until both sides of the bread was brown.

• 1/2 teaspoon granulated garlic

• 1/2 teaspoon kosher salt

1 teaspoon freshly ground black pepper

• Dijon mustard•

• 2 teaspoons.

• 1 **navel orange**

• Lemon juice

Bold = foods produced by bees

Have a look at this:

Preheat the oven to 375°F. 1.

1. Cook the pork in the oil 2.Drizzle the pork with the dried garlic

____. 4.Rub them in a small bowl with the balsamic glaze and salt. Let stand 5 minutes. 5.Remove from the grill, brush with the olive

Remove the skillet from the heat.

After combining the mustard and honey, add the mixture to the breaded pork chops. Blend well with a fork. 6. Toast the bread on a pan or on a griller. Serve the pork chops and top with the grilled bread.

(inserted) 6.Cut the orange completely into slices, with the flesh still attached to the skin. Using a peeler, cut the peel into thin strips and place them in the skillet.

7. Roast the pork in the oven for 10-15 minutes until it reaches a temperature of 145 degrees. Remove the meat from the oven and squeeze the lemon juice over it. Let it wait for at least 5 minutes.

Cut the tenderloins in diagonal slices and place slices of cooked orange on the plate. Serve sliced pork with pan drippings mixed in it. Oh my!

Roasted and Brussels Sprouts with Garlic

Serves 4–5

My mother didn't cook much from scratch, but she would often have cooked-in-the-bag vegetables. In fact, for vegetables, it's okay if you start them frozen since they are thawed in the microwave. Oven roasting is a better option, especially for root vegetables and sweet potatoes. Garlic helps as well, so massage a clove or two into sundry root vegetables before roasting, and then make broth as a by-product.

Roasting Brussels sprouts, the traditional way by baking them in an oven, is the best; however, you can prepare them as a side dish when you cook other foods.

The ingredients

1 stalk of Brussels sprouts.

• **garlic** is chopped into small pieces.

½ cup extra-virgin olive oil.

• 1 teaspoon salt.

"Bold" = "foods pollinated or produced by bees" (suggested by @randizik)

Here's what you do

Make sure the oven is heated up.

2. After preparing the sprouts, cut them in half so they remain flat on the baking sheet.

Spread the chopped garlic on the sprouts. Drizzle with olive oil, and sprinkle with salt.

4. Bake meatloaf in a oven that preheats to about 400°F for 20 to 25 hours. Afterward, taste it and add a bit more salt if desired.

5. 5.Serve immediately.

Citrus Smoothies

Serves 4–6

Fruit Smoothies are easy to make and are great for a breakfast or an afternoon snack. In season one, I accidentally made a version without ice. I found that when I replicated this ice-free smoothie, it was even better. Many blenders can produce ice cubes; you can even buy a special container for this purpose. If you don't, finely chop the ice before adding it to the smoothie.

The honey enhances the taste.

The ingredients:

- 1 medium banana
- Cut two or three tablespoons of strawberries.

Orange

- 2 cups plain yogurt
- • • • ½ cup **orange juice**

continue to...

- 1 teaspoon vanilla extract.

Saute the onions, but finely. Bring ½ cups cider, ½ cup brown sugar, and ½ cup ketchup to a boil and then add everything to

- 4-6 whole **strawberries** for garnish

Bold= foods that have bee pollinated= produce by bees.

What to do

1.Combine the banana, strawberries, orange zest, yogurt, orange juice, honey, vanilla, and ice in a blender and process for about 1 minute. You're done!

Put red strawberries into glasses and top each with a big dollop of whipped cream. Yum!

Coconut Macaroons with Dried Cherries

Makes 25–30 small cookies

I always thought macaroons were one of those rare treats that are overpriced and hard to find, but these; my friends, are easy. Use your favorite dried fruit, and the honey and butter drizzle adds a crispy edge to soft centers, and the tiny bit of salt balances the sweetness. Instead of melting chocolate in a bowl, dip each fluffy, crumbly bit of goodness halfway into it. What

The ingredients

us/no sweeteners Paraphrase: cup unsweetened flaked coconut

A time to celebrate

- 8 egg whites
- Salt
- 1/4 cup dried cherries
- 2 tablespoons butter

Honey is a great thing for your teeth.

Post a bold recipe

Here's what you do

Turn on the oven to 350 degrees Fahrenheit.

You should have a slide in coconut with sweetened coconut to the side. Heat and toast the coconut.

Reduce the oven temperature to 325°F.

4. To get the egg whites to stiffen up, salt is added to them until the whites turn into stiff peaks.

Mix 5.Fold into the egg white mixture. 5.Fold Coconut and Egg

You will make macarons by pouring tablespoon-sized rounds of coconut mixtures onto a parchment-lined baking sheet.

You may press one or two dried cherries into the top of each macaroon after baking.

Boil the butter and honey in the microwave for 20 seconds and drizzle the mixture onto the inside of each bite. Sprinkle with a tiny pinch of salt.

Bake for 40 minutes or for your oven's usual baking time, depending on how dry the weather is. Watch carefully as they bake to avoid burning. If you live in a dry climate, they will still taste crispy on the outside when you're done baking.

February

The properties of honey

The bee does not concern

The gardener, any time, to him

Is aristocracy.

— Emily Dickinson

Have a featured varietal

Tupelo Honey

Color: Moderate warm red.

Smell: Stewed fruit such as mangos, in the middle of floral scents.

The taste profile: Buttery, lightly caramelized

Aftertaste: None

Tupelo honey is similar to other honeys, such as clover and wildflower honey, but the bees are more selective about the nectar they choose to give the sweetness. The nectar is composed of sugars, enzymes, and natural growth factors. It's the waxy coating around that sugar that gives it its unique flavor and enables it to stick to your spoon without clumping.

's Leaneau's Grilled Pineapple Skewers

Makes 24 skewers

Lea brought some of her holiday mandelbrodt from her sailboat years with her into our dinner. I've adapted her Mediterranean dish with a different and interesting honey to celebrate all the delicious Thanksgivings we have had.

The ingredients

• • • • 3 **garlic** cloves, chopped 4 **garlic** cloves, chopped • **chillies</**

• One teaspoon of minced fresh ginger. Original: • Grated lemon rind 1 teaspoon minced fresh ginger Paraphrase: • Grated lemon rind

• 1/2 cup soy sauce.

• ¼ cup honey, preferred, is up to you.

• 2 tablespoons lime juice

Two tablespoons of white or sweet wine; or water.

1 Tablespoon Sesame Oil

• Cut 2 an Ace of Hearts card in half Paraphrase: Cut a medium-size round from an Ace of Hearts card.

The skewers can be cut to the length you want.

Bold = foods pollinated or produced by bees

Here are what you do

2.Combine the garlic, ginger, soy sauce, honey, lime juice, white wine and sesame oil in a medium-size non-reactive bowl. Stir well to combine. Add the chunks of pineapple and stir well, coating all the chunks with the marinade. Let sit for 1 hour, either

If electric or gas, the skewers should only be cooked for 4 minutes on one side but for 5 minutes on the other.

Slice the pineapple in half. Skewer it. Grill, then broil. For best results, broil the pineapple for about two (2) minutes per side. That would be two (2) minutes for each side of the pineapple.

If you want to prepare your food as quickly as possible, you may want to let your guests take skewers off of the grill.

Mama's Home-Style Winter Vegetable Soup

Serves 6–8

Ever since my grandmother died, my mother has adopted and adapted many of her grandmother's recipes. She introduced them to me early in life as well.

The vegetables used in this soup must be local and fresh. You can alter the vegetables based on seasonal availability. The soup improves with age.

The ingredients

• • • • • • • 4 medium **sweet onions**, peeled and cut into thin round slices 5

Carrots are good for you. Peel the carrots like the agent says. Done!

• 1 **turnip**, peeled and cut into ½-inch cubes

Leek should be washed and cut into 1-inch pieces.

1 cup of chopped celery, including the tops.

• 4 fresh curly **parsley** sprigs for garnishment.

1 teaspoon of salt.

• ½ cup French green beans (or green beans, cut into ½-inch pieces)

• 1/2 cup broccoli florets • 1/2 cup broccoli stems

• 1/2 cup **peas**

• Vegetables like bell peppers should be cut in slivers. -->

- 1 tablespoon butter
- ½ cup grated Parmesan or Grana Padano cheese

The bold <= italicized FOODS pollinated or produced by bees>

Here's what to do

1. 1.Combine the onions, carrots, turnip, leek, celery, and parsley in a large soup pot. Cover with about 2 quarts water and bring to a boil. Add the salt. Reduce the heat to a simmer. Cook until the vegetables are tender, 30 to 40 minutes.

Add the haricots verts and broccoli stems to the pot of boiling water and let them cook for 15 minutes.

Add the broccoli, peas, and bell pepper, and cook them until they are tender, about 15 minutes. Then, add the butter.

Ladle soup into bowls and garnish with Parmesan.

What's inside those beehives?

Factorymade beehives are designed to get rid of bees inside, and are made to be simple to care for. They are also designed to harvest honey as easily and as fast as possible.

You have probably seen cheese-stuffed doughnuts stacked in a field or on a roof or in a yard. At the bottom of the stack is the deepest box, which is called the "bucket body" or the "brood box." This is where

There are three types of supers available. The deep super is for the deepest honey comb. The medium and shallow supers are for the medium and shallow honeycomb.

The hive body is the super for bees storing honey and pollen, and if the hive is being raised for the queen's brood, then this is the super where the process is kept. For hive bodies with empty frames, the supers can be moved into different place.

A beekeeper must work with each bee to determine its intelligence. A shallow box of bees requires less physical strength than a larger super. I wouldn't be surprised to find that people have created puzzles, computers, and other fun gadgets out of nature. Scientists have reduced math and chemistry to the level of a game. Creationists call this taking God's nature out of His Creation.

Langstroth hives *(the most popular type) don't respect what is called "bee space." Bees love personal space and prefer ⅜ inch between their honeycombs. A wild honeybee colony will always have ⅜ inch of space between their honeycombs. Our Langstroth hives are the most popular hive and attempt to mimick what the bees do naturally.*

Curried Chicken with Coconut

Serves 8

This dish is one of my mom's recipes that I've adapted to be easier to eat. We make it a lot because it tastes so good. It is a nice dish to serve cold or at room temperature for a special occasion. You don't even have to cook it. If you want to make it ahead of time, you can freeze it, defrost, and serve when you have no energy to cook. The flavour really improves if you leave it for a few hours. This mild curry goes well with rice.

The ingredients

Chicken stock for the chicken and stock

- 2 **carrots**

*

1 cup chopped celery, with the tops. 2 tablespoons butter Paraphrase: 2 tablespoons butter. 3 onions, diced Paraphrase:

- 1 bay leaf
- 4 whole peppercorns
- 2 Tablespoons Salt

Parts of the boneless, skinless chicken like —

Get a coconut curry.

4 Tablespoons room temp unsalted butter.

- ½ cup unbleached all-purpose flour
- 2 **garlic** cloves

- 1½ tablespoons curry powder.
- ½ teaspoon paprika
- 1 tablespoon **honey**, your favorite honey
- ½ cup half-and-half
- ½ cup chopped unsweetened coconut

Bolded = special foods pollinated or produced by bees

Here are the things you need to do

1. Acquire 1 quart of water. Add 1/3 cup of carrots, 1 inch of onions, 1 stalk of celery, a bay leaf, a few peppercorns, and a bit of salt. Bring to a boil. Add the chicken to the pot, then reduce the heat to a simmer and

Place the chicken in a large pot with 4 quarts of cold water, 1 cup of chicken stock, and 3 bay leaves. Bring the water to a boil, then reduce the heat to medium. Lower the heat even more when the water becomes fragrant and turns a dull orange. Let simmer for 1 hour or more until the chicken is quite tender. Remove from heat, cover with a lid, and let let cool.

Pick off the meat and discard the bones. Bring the broth back up to a boil and cook the meat in it for another 30. Remove the meat from the broth, and refrigerate it if you will not be completing the recipe.

4. Mix one-quarter cup of the stock with the olive oil in a bowl. When you are ready to complete the recipes, just pour in the remaining stock and blend until the soup is completely smooth.

To prepare the coconut curry, melt the butter in a large skillet over medium-low heat. Turn the heat down to low when the butter has melted.

Add the flour and pulse in a food processor until slightly mixed. At this point, add the garlic, curry powder, paprika, and honey and blend well, making sure that the paprika and honey are spread evenly throughout.

When making a hot *half-and-half*, begin by slowly stirring a few cups of the stock. You want your sauce to be smooth and nicely thick until it's like *honey*.

8.To fold in the reserved chicken and coconut just before serving, starting with the membrane. If the consistency is too thick for you, then add more stock.

9. Add to your dinner as much as you like of the coconut.

Measuring Honey

You may also want to deposit a few drops of liquid petroleum jelly on the spoon or cup first. The honey will then spread out easily.

Sweet and Salty Kale Crisps

Serves 2–3 as a side. It's also good as a cocktail-hour nibble.

This kale recipe is easy to make and tastes great with a touch of honey. One of my farmer friends suggests that I spritz the leaves with olive oil and bake them until crisp and golden brown. I recently wondered what would happen if I added a little sweetness to the mix. This dessert combines flavors, giving me a sweet, bitter, salty, and sour taste all in one bite.

The components

• 2–3 tablespoons extra-virgin olive oil • 1 bunch curly kale (you may also use other types of kale; have fun experimenting)

• a quarter teaspoon of kosher salt

• 1/8 teaspoon black pepper, freshly ground

• 1 tablespoon honey (tupelo honey preferred)

• 1 tablespoon vinegar (red wine)

Bee pollinated or produced foods are bolded.

Here's how it works:

1. Preheat the oven to 350 degrees Fahrenheit.

2. Separate the leaves from the stems of the kale. Fill your compost bucket with the stems. Any large leaves should be ripped into 2 to 3 inch pieces.

3. Spray the torn leaves with olive oil and arrange them on a baking sheet. (I store olive oil in a spray bottle similar to that which is used to spritz plants.) If you don't have a spray bottle, combine the kale and oil in a bowl before spreading on the baking sheet. Add salt and pepper to taste.

4. 4.Bake for 20 minutes, stirring once or twice, until crisp. Remove the kale from the oven, drizzle with honey, and bake for another 5 minutes. Remove the leaves from the oven and drizzle with the red wine vinegar.

5. Serve right away, allowing visitors to serve themselves to the crispy finger food.

Fresh Fruit and Israeli Couscous

Serves 8

Cooking and eating Israeli couscous is a lot of fun. Unlike conventional couscous, which has tiny completed grains, Israeli couscous cooks into small, smooth, spherical beads. In my café, we frequently serve this salad at room temperature, but it can also be served warm. Another significant benefit is that it cooks rapidly and is an excellent starch. If you're preparing this in the dead of winter, feel free to add freshly roasted seasonal veggies and fresh herbs from your garden or windowsill.

The components

- 1 tsp. salt
- 1 cup couscous from Israel (also called pearl couscous)
- 14 cup tamari almonds, sliced
- a quarter cup of raisins
- 1 peeled orange, cut into pieces
- 1 scallion, thinly sliced
- a quarter cup of extra-virgin olive oil
- 2 tbsp apple cider vinegar

Bee pollinated or produced foods are bolded.

Here's how it works:

1. In a small saucepan, bring 114 cups lightly salted water to a boil. Stir in the couscous, cover, and reduce the heat to a low simmer. Cook, stirring occasionally, for 5 to 8 minutes, or until the water has been absorbed. Allow to cool after removing the saucepan from the heat.

2. In a 1-quart mixing basin, combine the couscous, almonds, raisins, orange pieces, and scallion. Toss the salad with the olive oil and vinegar. Enjoy!

Bananas Baked with Honeyed Cream

Serves 8

Baked bananas were a staple in my childhood. Although we were not a dessert-loving family, this meal was frequently served at our table, especially on cold winter nights. Just thinking about it makes me feel warm. In the creamy sauce, my mother used brown sugar as the sweetener, but I prefer honey now. Tupelo honey complements the cream and adds a subtle sweetness to the bananas.

The components

• 4 bananas (ripe)

• 4 tablespoons salted butter, cubed

2 tsp. light brown sugar

• 1 orange juice cup

1 quart sour cream

• 1 tablespoon honey (tupelo honey preferred)

• 1 tsp. vanilla extract

Bee pollinated or produced foods are bolded.

Here's how it works:

1. Preheat the oven to 375 degrees Fahrenheit.

2. Peel and cut the bananas in half lengthwise. Place the bananas in a pretty baking dish that can be taken to the table. Sprinkle with brown sugar and a dot of butter.

3. Carefully pour the orange juice into the baking dish's bottom, being careful not to disturb the butter and sugar.

Bake for 15 minutes, or until the bananas are gently browned and the liquid in the bottom of the dish is bubbling. Allow to cool slightly after removing from the oven.

5. 5.In a small mixing bowl, combine the sour cream, honey, and vanilla extract.

6. Arrange the baking dish on the table with the bowl of sour cream sauce on the side. Allow guests to self-serve by taking half a banana, some juice, and a dollop of the sauce.

Slushes of Mango–Key Lime

Serves 6–8

This is a really refreshing beverage. The key lime juice adds a subtle and unusual background flavour that is far more interesting than conventional lime juice. If you can't find fresh key limes, you can generally get the juice, already squeezed, near the cocktail mixing area in your grocery store (near the cherries and olives and fancy stirrers). Make sure the mangos are really ripe and sweet for the finest results.

I recommend pineapple mint as a mint garnish because it is extremely wonderful and complements the tastes in this cocktail, though chocolate mint may also be fun. If these types are unavailable, ordinary mint will suffice.

The components

- 3 cups mango chunks
- 1 orange juice cup
- key lime juice (13 cup)
- 14 cup honey (tupelo honey preferred)
- a quarter teaspoon of salt
- ice cubes, 4–5 cups
- Garnish with fresh mint sprigs

Bee pollinated or produced foods are bolded.

Here's how it works:

1. In a blender, combine the mango, orange juice, key lime juice, honey, and salt. Pulse until everything is well combined and puréed.
2. 2.Pulse in the ice cubes until the mixture resembles an icy blend. With a decent, vigorous blender, this will take 10 to 15 seconds. In roughly 5 seconds, a Vitamix mixer will do the trick.
3. 3.Serve in glasses with a sprig of fresh mint as a garnish. Serve right away.

March

I see the cautious bug among his works.

The delicious dew has now been exhausted from the blooms;

His small thighs are laden with golden jewels.

And guide him across the heavens on his long trek.

— "Rural sports," by John Gay

Tasting Notes for Featured Varietals

Honey from Acacia

Light yellow in colour

Very mild odour

Taste: Buttery vanilla with a subtle, fresh flavour.

Aftertaste: Caramel is very subtle and sweet.

Acacia honey is prepared from the blossoms of the false acacia tree, often known as the black locust tree in the United States. This tree, which is endemic to the northeastern United States, is well-known throughout Europe.

Acacia honey can be found in speciality shops here. It is mostly made in Bulgaria, Hungary, and Romania, but it is also widely available in France and Italy. Pick some up when you're on the road or in a specialty honey shop! It'll be the lightest honey you've ever had, and it'll go great with your morning tea, toast, or any of the recipes in this chapter. Acacia honey is also known for being one of the greatest wound-healing honeys.

Dilled Cream Dipping Sauce for Roasted Baby Vegetables

This appetiser serves 8 people.

Early spring is the best time to go grocery shopping for the freshest baby vegetables. We're a little too far north in Asheville to grow our own fruit, but we do have regional vegetables in our supermarkets, which I like to roast with coarse salt and serve with a delicious herbed dip to my friends. Although this dish does not contain honey, honeybees pollinate all of the veggies listed. Honeybees, thank you.

Tell your guests about the "every third bite" story that inspired your selection (see page 9) and your presentation will rise beyond the standard veggie tray. If you cook this in a different season, see the list on page 195 for alternative veggies you can use.

The components

Regarding the vegetables

- 1 pound of baby carrots, entire if possible, with tops removed
- 1 bunch (about 1 pound) baby beets, tops removed but 1 inch of stem left
- 1 bunch (1 pound) baby turnips, tops removed but 1 inch of stem left
- a quarter cup of extra-virgin olive oil

• 1 bunch (12 pound) radishes, tops trimmed but 1 inch of stalk remaining

• 12 pound fresh peas (optional)

In order to make the dipping sauce

• 2 cups Greek yoghurt, plain

• 1 tablespoon dill (fresh)

• 1 lime, zest

• 1 lime's juice

• Sea salt

Bee pollinated or produced foods are bolded.

Here's how it works:

1. Preheat the oven to 375 degrees Fahrenheit.

2. Slice any carrots longer than 4 inches into 2-inch-long diagonal slices.

3. Cut any large beets or turnips into little pieces.

4. Toss the carrots, beets, and turnips in the olive oil separately and spread out on a large baking sheet, keeping the vegetables separated. Bake for 20 to 30 minutes (less time for small vegetables), watching frequently toward the end to ensure they don't burn. Tender but not excessively soft vegetables are ideal. Allow time for cooling.

5. Slice any large radishes into little pieces.

6. 6.If using peas that aren't quite fresh, bring a small pot of water to a boil and immerse them in it for 2 minutes, or until they turn bright green. To halt the cooking and retain them bright green, remove them and quickly plunge them into a bowl of icy water. If the peas are truly fresh, don't cook them.

7. 7.In a medium mixing bowl, combine the yoghurt, dill, lime zest, and lime juice. Season with a pinch or two of salt.

Place the vegetables on a serving plate and serve. I prefer to build small mounds of each object and arrange them in colour order (red, orange, yellow, green, blue, indigo, and violet), although a random scatter is as entertaining. I like to utilise something from the dish as garnish, so I sometimes use the tops of the vegetables as a foundation or to tuck around the dip bowl.

Interesting Fact

1 pound of beeswax is made up of 500,000 wax flakes.

Rhubarb Soup by Elsie

Serves 8–10

Readers and visitors to Blueberry Hill Inn sent my mother their favourite dishes after she published The Blueberry Hill Cookbook and the inn became more popular. Many of these become favourites of ours. This is one of them. Recipe is one of my favourites now that it has been adjusted to include honey instead of sugar, despite the fact that it is uncommon. You may think of it as a dessert soup. Buy some rhubarb and cook this soup as soon as it pokes up enough to cut or as soon as it comes in your markets.

The egg yolk thickens the soup in this dish. Leave out the raw egg if you're afraid of it, but I'm confident using a fresh, local, organic egg.

The components

• 3 cups rhubarb, thinly sliced (in a pinch, it is okay to use frozen as long as it is plain frozen rhubarb)

• 1 tblsp cornstarch

• 12 cup honey, preferably acacia or the lightest local honey available

12 cup whipping cream, chilled

• 1 egg yolk (organic)

• 1 lemon zest for garnish

Bee pollinated or produced foods are bolded.

Here's how it works:

1. In a medium, nonreactive saucepan, cover the rhubarb with cold water and bring to a boil. Cook, stirring occasionally, until the fruit is very soft, perhaps 15 minutes or more.

2. 2.Rhubarb should be pressed through a sieve or, better yet, a food mill. This will keep the rhubarb's rough, stringy portions out of the soup. Throw the strings in the garbage. Return to the saucepan with the rhubarb mixture.

3. 3.In a small cup, whisk together the cornstarch and 14 cup cool water. Stir the cornstarch into the rhubarb mixture until it is completely clear (from the cornstarch mixture).

4. 4.Toss the cornstarch and rhubarb mixture with the honey. If the rhubarb is particularly tart, add a little more honey, but not too much. This soup is notable for its lack of sweetness. Chill completely.

5. 5.In a medium mixing bowl, whip the chilled cream and egg yolk until firm peaks form (be careful not to produce butter!). Add to the soup and mix thoroughly.

6. Serve with lemon zest as a garnish.

Salad with Mushrooms and Dill

Serves 4–5

This recipe is fantastic! It's ideal for a springtime luncheon or as a side dish for a spring dinner. It's ideal if you make it a few hours ahead of time. Sugar was used in the original recipe.

March's varietal, acacia honey, has supplanted it, adding a delicious richness and complexity that is far more interesting. Give this one a shot.

The components

- button mushrooms, 1 pound
- 1 tablespoon curly parsley, chopped, plus extra for garnish
- 1 tablespoon salt
- celery seeds (12 teaspoon)
- 12 teaspoon coarsely chopped fresh dill
- 1/8 teaspoon garlic granules
- 1 gallon heavy cream
- 1 lemon's zest
- 1 lemon's juice (about 2 tablespoons)
- 12 teaspoon honey (acacia honey is preferred)
- 1 Bibb lettuce head

Bee pollinated or produced foods are bolded.

Here's how it works:

1. If the mushroom stems' bottoms are soiled, trim them off. Thinly slice the mushrooms into "umbrella" slices.

2. 2.In a 1-quart mixing basin, whisk together the mushrooms, parsley, salt, celery seeds, dill, garlic, heavy cream, lemon zest, lemon juice, and honey until the mushrooms are well coated in the cream mixture.

3. 3.If feasible, chill for at least 1 hour.

4. Arrange a few lettuce leaves on each salad plate and top each with 1 cup of mushrooms. Serve with additional parsley as a garnish.

In a bee colony, there are three types of bees: the queen, the drones, and the workers. The colony is led by the queen. Bees can survive without a queen, but the hive will not be able to grow and thrive without her.

The queen's major function is to lay eggs, which she does all day, every day, throughout the warm seasons. She can lay up to 1,500 eggs every day, which weigh more than she does when tallied. She is the only bee capable of laying eggs that will hatch into colony members.

She is the colony's largest bee and is pretty easy to recognise. She is frequently surrounded by a small group of people who groom, feed, and look after her. The queen has a distinct scent, known as a pheromone, which is disseminated throughout the colony by the workers, indicating to all bees that she is their leader and that this is their home.

Although some beekeepers believe she stops being productive after two years, the queen has an effective life span of up to five years. Those beekeepers either produce a new queen or purchase one from a breeder to replace her. When worker bees notice that their queen has left or is not performing well, they will “create” a new queen.

Worker bees will develop a new, spacious cell for a few eggs to “make” a new queen. When other workers notice the enlarged queen cell, they will feed the eggs “royal jelly,” a rich nourishment that other bee infants enjoy for a brief time but the queen gets for much longer. Unfortunately, this is a survival of the fittest situation: the first queen to hatch will destroy the others. If more than one hatches by chance, the strongest one wins and assumes control of the hive.

A newborn queen spends her first few days within the hive before taking “mating flights,” which are brief ventures into the air near the hive. The queen connects and mates with a number of drones from other colonies in what are known as “drone assembly zones” (I think of them as bee singles bars). The queen mates with an average of 12 distinct drones over the course of a day or two, absorbing their genetic material. When she returns to her home hive following her mating flights, she spends the rest of her life within the hive, laying genetically varied eggs.

Chapter Two

THE RECIPES

Roasted Whole Chicken with Fresh Herbs

Serves 4–6

My sister gave me a fancy replacement for baking a chicken over a beer can: a ceramic chicken baker. The chicken made from beer cans is delicious, while the paint from the cans isn't. However, I digress. This chicken recipe is suitable for Passover, Easter, spring, or any other supper, and it does not require the use of a special baker. Here is my recommendation for you.

The components

- 1 (3–4 pound) farm-fresh chicken
- 2 cut-in-half lemons
- 2 medium sweet onions (cut into large wedges)
- 6 peeled garlic cloves
- 4 rosemary sprigs, fresh

- 4 sprigs fresh thyme
- Baby potatoes, 1 pound
- 2 peeled carrots, cut into 1-inch diagonal slices
- 2 celery stalks, sliced diagonally into 1-inch slices
- 1 tablespoon salt
- 1 teaspoon black pepper, freshly ground
- 1 teaspoon garlic granules
- 2 tblsp unsalted butter, sliced into cubes
- 2 tbsp honey (ideally acacia honey)

Bee pollinated or produced foods are bolded.

Here's how it works:

1. Preheat the oven to 375 degrees Fahrenheit.

2. Remove the giblets from the chicken and wash it (you can use them for stock later, if you like). Place the chicken in a deep roasting pan after drying it (a 13-inch pan is good).

3. 3.In the cavity of the bird, tuck the halves of 1 lemon, the slices of 1 onion, 2 garlic cloves, and 2 rosemary and thyme sprigs each. Scatter the remaining onion, the remaining 4 garlic cloves, the potatoes, carrots, and celery in the bottom of the roaster. Cut the potatoes in half if they are larger than bite-size.

4. 4.Salt, pepper, and granulated garlic season the chicken. Spread the butter on the bird.

5. 5.Bake for 112 hours, or until the juices run clear when a small knife is inserted where the leg and the body meet. You may need to alter the time if your chicken is larger or your oven is slower than mine.

6. Allow at least 15 minutes for the chicken to rest before chopping. The fluids will stay in the meat rather than flowing out into the pan. Drizzle the honey over the chicken while it's resting.

7. Arrange the cooked veggies on a dish and top with the chicken, whole or sliced up. Garnish with the remaining 2 rosemary and thyme sprigs. Serve by squeezing the remaining lemon halves over the plate and pouring any pan juices on top.

Citrus Punch with Sparkle

Approximately 20 people

We make this punch for gatherings all the time. It's simple, refreshing, and versatile. Play around with it to suit the season and your preferences. Reconstituted unsweetened frozen juice will suffice if you don't have fresh squeezed juice. If you're using frozen concentrates, use two parts water instead of the suggested three.

If you don't have an ice mould, simply fill the punch bowl halfway with ice and top with fresh fruit slices. This punch is extremely appealing because of the fresh fruit pieces.

The components

1 lemon (cut into rings)

1 lime (cut into rings)

1 orange (cut into rings)

- 20 strawberries, whole (optional)
- As needed, ice cubes
- 1 bottle ginger ale (2 litres)
- 2 lemon juice glasses
- 1 gallon orange juice
- 1 lime juice cup
- 14 cup fresh mint leaves, entire

Bee pollinated or produced foods are bolded.

Here's how it works:

1. Fill a ring mould halfway with lemon, lime, and orange slices, as well as the strawberries, if using, the day before the party. Fill the mould with cold water and more fruit to fill it. Fill the mould with the fruit in your sink to prevent excess water from

spilling out. Transfer to the freezer with care (putting it on a baking sheet helps) and freeze altogether.

2. Fill a big punch bowl halfway with ice cubes just before your guests arrive. In a punch bowl, combine the ginger ale, lemon juice, orange juice, and lime juice.

3. 3.To remove the ice ring, run the outside of the mould under hot water for a few seconds to encourage the ice to slide out. In the punch bowl, place the mould. It will slowly melt as it floats in the punch, allowing the fruit to float. So lovely!

4. 4.Add the mint leaves as a garnish.

Tzimmes

Serves 4

There are several different varieties of this traditional Jewish food. And, because it's a dish that takes a long time to prepare and requires a lot of washing, peeling, chopping, and other labour, the word tzimmes has evolved to mean "a huge deal."

Despite the fact that I am Jewish (my mother is), we did not grow up in a traditional Jewish family or with this food. Nonetheless, I've grown to enjoy it as a side dish to a relaxing, comforting dinner of roasted chicken. It's a traditional Passover dish, but it's also a fantastic addition to any cold-weather feast. Don't let the "big deal" scare you. Making this one is not difficult.

The components

- 1 pound carrots, peeled and cut diagonally into 1-inch slices
- 1 pound peeled sweet potatoes, cut into 1-inch chunks
- 12 pound Yukon Gold potatoes, cubed to 1 inch
- 12 cup cut-in-half dried apricots

12 cup prunes, pitted and chopped in half

- 1/8 teaspoon cinnamon powder
- 1 lemon's zest
- 1 lemon's juice
- 2 tbsp. butter (cut into bits)
- 14 cup honey (ideally acacia honey) plus a little extra for dripping
- 14 cup almond slivers
- 1 teaspoon salt (kosher or sea)
- black pepper, freshly ground

Bee pollinated or produced foods are bolded.

Here's how it works:

1. Preheat the oven to 350 degrees Fahrenheit.

2. 2.In a large soup pot, combine the carrots, sweet potatoes, and Yukon Gold potatoes and cover with lukewarm water. Cook for about 15 minutes, or until the vegetables are starting to get soft.

3. 3.Using a slotted spoon, transfer the veggies to a baking dish and scatter the apricots and prunes about the vegetables. Cinnamon, lemon zest, and lemon juice are sprinkled over top. Butter the mixture and sprinkle the honey over everything.

4. Bake for 30 minutes, covered with aluminium foil. Remove the foil, sprinkle the almonds on top, and bake for another 10 minutes, or until a fork slips easily through the vegetables. Before serving, season with salt and pepper to taste, as well as a drizzle of honey.

Panna Cotta with Kumquats Candied

Serves 6

Anything with custard, cream, or custard cream in it is the most comfortable of comfort foods for me. Panna cotta, which translates as “cooked cream” in Italian, is at the top of my list of comfort foods. Adapt the basic recipe as needed. I’ve had a delightful lemony version floating on a light cucumber soup, a cheesy version served with a midsummer corn chowder, and a Cointreau-infused version served as a light finish to a winter feast. This dish was created in response to a new crop of kumquats.

The components

To make the panna cotta, combine all of the ingredients in a mixing bowl.

- 1 gallon whole milk
- 1 tablespoon gelatin powder, unflavored
- 3 cups heavy cream
- 13 cup honey (acacia preferred)
- 1 tsp. salt

For the kumquats candied

- 12 cup honey (acacia honey is preferred)
- 4 cups kumquats, sliced and seeded (sliced in half)

Bee pollinated or produced foods are bolded.

Here's how it works:

1. To create the panna cotta, pour the milk into a small mixing bowl and stir in the gelatin until smooth. Allow approximately 5 minutes for the gelatin to soften.

2. 2.Pour the mixture into a small heavy saucepan and cook over medium heat for 5 minutes, or until the gelatin has dissolved. Make sure the milk doesn't boil.

3. Remove from the heat and mix in the cream, honey, and salt. Pour into six glasses, small bowls, or cups for serving. Allow it cool completely before refrigerating for 6 hours.

4. In a small nonreactive saucepan, combine 12 cup water and the honey to prepare the kumquats. Stir thoroughly and bring to a boil, stirring occasionally. Return to a boil with the kumquats, then lower to a low heat and cook until the kumquats are soft, about 15 to 20 minutes. Cook for another 5 minutes, or until the liquid has reduced to a thick syrup. Allow to cool to room temperature after removing from the heat.

5. Spoon the kumquats over the panna cotta to serve.

Dark brown colour of avocado honey

Warm vegetal scent; hayfield

Taste: Molasses, burned sugar

Aftertaste: Cane syrup lingers

Avocado blossom nectar is used to make avocado honey. Avocados are most commonly grown in California, but they can also be found in warm climates such as Florida and the Southwest. Avocado honey, on the other hand, has nothing in common with avocados. Avocado nectar turns into a dark, thick honey that tastes like molasses, sorghum, or Louisiana-style cane syrup. Avocado honey will complement any of these sweeteners, as well as dark brown sugar, in recipes.

Bees produce avocado honey while pollinating citrus trees, mustard plants, and other blooming trees in the growing area. Honeybees prefer citrus flowers because they have a richer fragrance. As a result, pure avocado honey is a unique honey that can only be found in hives near avocado trees.

Guacamole of Choice

Serves 4

I adore guacamole, and I rarely leave the house without a pair of Hass avocados, the ones with the black rippling skin. The avocado is ripe and ready when the peel yields to light pressure. You don't need to do much to produce delicious guacamole if the avocado is ripe. There is no honey in this dish, but I included it because avocados would not exist without bees.

The components

- avocados (two)
- 1 little sliced ripe tomato
- 1 scallion (white and green sections) sliced into thin rings
- 2 tablespoons fresh cilantro, finely chopped
- 1 lime, zest

- 1 lime's juice
- Sea salt, coarse
- 1 tablespoon jalapeo, minced (optional)
- 1 large bag of salted tortilla chips (about 16 ounces)

Bee pollinated or produced foods are bolded.

Here's how it works:

1. Remove the pits from the avocados and cut them in half. (I nick the pit with the knife blade, turn it quickly to release the pit from the flesh, then lift my knife blade with the pit stuck to it.) The pit can be removed with a swift smack on the edge of a plastic compost bucket.)

2. Scoop the flesh into a medium bowl with a spoon and mash with a fork, pausing while the avocado is still chunky.

3. Combine the tomato, scallion, cilantro, lime zest, and lime juice in a large mixing bowl. Stir carefully, making sure the mixture remains chunky. Season with salt to taste. Add the jalapeo if you like things hot.

4. Toss with tortilla chips and serve.

Browning and How to Avoid It

If you're not serving the guacamole right away, leave the avocado pit in the serving bowl to keep the guacamole from browning. Remove the pit just before serving.

Salad with Avocado and Mango

As a side dish, it serves 4 people.

My café has been blessed with cooks from all around the United States and perhaps the world throughout the years. This fast salad is delicious and comes from El Salvador.

The components

- 1 avocado
- 1 mango, chopped into 12-inch cubes
- 1 tiny lime zest
- 1 tiny lime juice
- 1 teaspoon fresh dill, coarsely chopped
- 1 teaspoon fresh cilantro leaves, entire (compost the stems)
- Sea salt
- Leaves of Bibb lettuce

Bee pollinated or produced foods are bolded.

Here's how it works:

1. Remove the pit from the avocado and cut it in half. While the flesh is still in its skin, cut it into 12-inch cubes. Using a tiny rubber spatula, gently separate the cubes from the skin and place them in a medium basin. Note: If you're careful, the avocado pieces will keep their cube shape, but don't worry if any get mashed. It will still be delicious.

2. 2. Season the mango cubes with lime zest, lime juice, dill, and cilantro. Season with salt to taste.

3. Place lettuce leaves on a dish and top with the avocado-mango combination.

Crème Fraîche Borscht

Serves 4

When you're in the market, get a lot of baby beets. Here's a wonderful, simple soup to cook with them - a great way to start the season, even if you don't like beets.

Make the crème fraîche at least 24 hours ahead of time.

The components

When it comes to the crème fraîche,

2 quarts thick cream

2 quarts sour cream

To make the borscht

- 1 pound of baby beets, tops removed
- 1 pound newly harvested potatoes
- 12 cup honey, avocado honey preferred
- Sea salt
- Dill leaves for garnish (optional)

Bee pollinated or produced foods are bolded.

Here's how it works:

1. In a jar, combine the heavy cream and sour cream to produce the crème fraîche. Shake well to combine, then set aside in a warm location overnight. (I use the refrigerator's top.) Refrigerate the cream once it has thickened until ready to use. Crème fraîche keeps for a week in the refrigerator.

2. 2.Cut the tops off the beets and cut them. In a 6-quart soup pot, combine the beets, chopped tops, and potatoes, then cover with about 2 quarts cold water. (Do not totally fill the saucepan; just cover the vegetables with water.) Bring to a boil, then turn down to a low heat. Cook for 15 to 20 minutes, depending on the size of the beets, until they can be punctured with a fork.

3. Fill a large basin halfway with ice water to create an ice bath. Using a slotted spoon, remove the beets and potatoes from the simmering liquid. Remove the skins from the cooked beets

and place them in an ice bath. Using a strainer or colander, strain the cooking liquid into a bowl. Cooked beet greens and beet skins should be composted.

4. Return the beets and potatoes to the soup, grated or chopped. Season with salt to taste after adding the honey.

5. 5.Serve each portion with 1 tablespoon crème fraîche. If desired, garnish with a sprinkling of fresh dill.

Bees that work

The workers are the most fascinating bees in the colony to me. They are in charge in many ways. The employees' jobs fluctuate throughout their life, unlike the queen and the drones, who each have one major duty.

All female worker bees begin working as housekeeping bees as soon as they are born. They clean out their birth cell as they emerge, preparing it for another egg from the queen. They quickly become undertakers, assisting in the removal of deceased bees from the hive. They are nurse bees from the age of three to eleven days, caring for newly placed eggs and larvae.

From days 12 to 17, the staff serve as queen attendants, looking after Her Majesty's feeding and grooming needs. The staff keep the queen at a steady temperature of 95 degrees Fahrenheit (35 degrees Celsius) all year, fanning her in the hotter months and clustering her in the cooler months. The queen attendants pick up her aroma (her pheromone) as they care for her and disseminate it to the other bees as they travel throughout the hive.

After that, the workers transform into house bees, who greet the foragers (more on them later), collect pollen and nectar, and store it in the hive. The house bees fan the watery nectar to get the right consistency of honey, build and maintain honeycomb, and keep the hive at the right temperature.

Workers begin to take duties outside the hives about 18 days after they are born, the first being guard bee. These bees linger around the hive's entrance, ensuring that no one who does not belong, as evidenced by their foreign aroma, enters.

The worker bee eventually evolves into a forager, gathering pollen and nectar and returning it to the hive. Scout bees go out first, looking for food sources and then returning to the hive. They execute a waggle dance, wriggling their bodies in a given way for a specific amount of time, to tell their sisters where to go. The direction they are facing shows the location of their discovery. The distance to the target is indicated by the length of the dance.

Baby Carrots Glazed

Serves 4

Put this meal on your dinner menu when you can harvest carrots right out of the ground. If you don't have access to a garden, look for fresh baby carrots at your local farmers' market. The produce area of your grocery store is the next choice. Instead of the packaged "baby" carrots, use small ordinary carrots. The better, the fresher they are.

The components

• 2 bunches entire baby carrots (approximately 1 pound), tops removed, sliced into 12-inch slices

• 1 tablespoon butter (unsalted)

• 1 tsp honey (ideally avocado honey)

• 1 tablespoon lemon juice, freshly squeezed

• Sea salt

Bee pollinated or produced foods are bolded.

Here's how it works:

1. In a large nonreactive pot, place the carrots. Bring to a boil with enough water to cover the bottom of the saucepan. Reduce to a low heat, cover, and cook for 5 minutes or less, just long enough to cook the carrots to an al dente texture. (I only cook them for a few minutes to warm them up.) Because baby carrots are so soft, they do not require much cooking. Except for kids, no one I know enjoys mushy carrots!)

2. 2.Return the carrots to the pot and stir in the butter. To melt the butter, return to the heat. Toss in the carrots with the honey and lemon juice.

3. Season with salt to taste and serve.

Nonreactive Saucepans are Essential

A nonreactive saucepan is one that is constructed of stainless steel, glass, ceramic, or is Teflon-coated. It's vital to remember that it won't react with acids (like lemon or vinegar). Reactive pans include those made of cast iron and aluminium.

Coffee with Avocado Honey Crust Rack of Lamb

Serves 4 (2 chops per person)

This is a variation of a popular Blueberry Hill dish. My mother used coffee to baste a brown sugar and mustard crust on a roast leg of lamb for special occasions. This is how I like to make it using dark avocado honey.

The components

- 14 cup freshly toasted bread crumbs
- 14 cup honey, avocado honey preferred
- 1 tablespoon coarse-ground mustard
- 1 rack of lamb, small (about 2 pounds)
- Sea salt

- Black pepper, coarsely ground
- Garlic granules
- 1 cup espresso or strong brewed coffee
- a quarter-cup of white wine

Bee pollinated or produced foods are bolded.

Here's how it works:

1. Preheat the oven to 375 degrees Fahrenheit.

2. 2.In a small bowl, add the bread crumbs, honey, and mustard and whisk until barely mixed.

3. 3.Salt, pepper, and granulated garlic season the lamb rack. On the meat side of the rack, spread the honey-mustard paste. Place the lamb rack in a baking dish just big enough to accommodate it, preferably one that can also be used on the stove. Pour the coffee into the baking dish's bottom.

4. Bake for 10 minutes, or until the crust is golden brown, then baste with the pan drippings, being careful not to dissolve the honey-mustard mixture. Bake for another 20 minutes or until a meat thermometer reaches 130°F. Keep a close eye on things. This may take less time if your racks are small. Larger racks will also take longer. Remove the pan from the oven after it has achieved the desired temperature. While you make the sauce, place the lamb rack on a warm dish to rest.

5.Preheat the oven and place the baking dish on top of it. Over medium-high heat, deglaze the pan with the wine, swirling constantly with a wooden spoon. Add any additional juices from the resting lamb that have accumulated on the platter. Stir for about 5 minutes, or until the drippings and wine are fully combined and somewhat thickened.

6. 6. Slice the rack into rib sections and serve with the warm sauce.

Crumbs of fresh bread

Simply cut a few slices of bread into tiny bits or pulse a few slices in a food processor for a few seconds to generate fresh bread crumbs. You're hoping for coarse crumbs rather than sand grains. To toast, put the bread in a dry saucepan over medium heat for a few minutes, or until golden brown.

Iced Tea, Southern Style

Serves 4

I moved to the South after growing up in the North, where iced tea was only a summertime beverage. Tea (presumably "iced") is a year-round beverage in North Carolina. I've become accustomed to it. My honeyed version is below. By the way, if you have enough sun in your location to create "sun tea" (by putting tea bags in a glass jar filled with water and letting it rest in the sun for a few hours), simply add honey while the water is still warm and you'll have delicious sweet honey tea in no time.

The components

1. 6 tea bags

2. 14–12 cup honey, avocado honey preferred (depending on how sweet you like your tea)

3. Garnish with fresh mint sprigs

Here's how it works:

1. Bring four cups of water to a boil. Fill a heatproof pitcher halfway with boiling water, then add the tea bags. Add the honey while the tea is still hot.

Allow for a 20-minute steep to make a strong tea. Tea bags should be removed.

3. 3.Reduce to room temperature or, better yet, prepare ahead of time and chill until ready to serve.

Pour the rich sweet tea into ice-filled glasses to serve. Garnish with sprigs of mint.

Cream of Strawberry-Rhubarb

Serves 6–8

In the spring, my mother prepared rhubarb cream, and I still make it using spears from a plant I received when I moved into my log cabin. Because rhubarb does not require bee pollination, I added strawberries to this dish, which do. Strawberries and rhubarb go along beautifully. This recipe is similar to a fruit pie, but it doesn't include the crust.

The components

• rhubarb stalks, 1 pound, sliced into 12-inch chunks

• 1 pound chopped strawberries

• 14 cup honey, avocado honey preferred (more or less to taste)

1 cup whipping cream, cooled

Bee pollinated or produced foods are bolded.

Here's how it works:

1. In a large nonreactive saucepan, combine the rhubarb and 1 cup water. Bring to a boil, then turn down to a low heat. Cook, stirring regularly, until the rhubarb is fork-tender, about 10 minutes.

2. Cook for another 5 minutes after adding 34 pounds of strawberries and the honey. Turn off the heat.

3. Mash the fruit mixture coarsely. If the rhubarb is particularly tart, add extra honey to taste. Chill.

4. Whip the cooled cream until it forms soft peaks. Whip the cream and fold it into the cold fruit mixture. Chill for at least an hour. (This might be made late in the afternoon for dinner later that evening.)

5. 5.Garnish with the remaining 14 pound strawberry slices in individual bowls.

Raspberry Honey is a light brown colour.

Woodsy scent

Taste: Brown sugar and toffee with a secondary note of bitterness

Finish: A light raspberry finish

With the exception of the northern Plains States, raspberry honey is made from the nectar of raspberry flowers produced primarily in the northern tier of the United States. The exquisite delicacy of the white blossom aroma fills the spring air.

Raspberry honey is light amber to light brown in colour and has a mild to medium woodsy and caramelised aroma. It has a subtle sweetness that reminds me of toffee or brown sugar. Vanilla, Champagne, chocolate, and fresh pears or peaches are also good choices.

Soup with Fresh Peas with Minted Cream

Serves 12

Mint and peas go well together, and this soup is a lovely spring appetiser. Instead of making a minty pea soup base, I like to sprinkle a mildly sweet, lightly lemony cream on top. This soup is made using fresh spring peas, but if you can't find them at the market or, better yet, from your garden, you may use frozen peas. Peas simmer rapidly, so if you come over some fresh peas, you may make this soup on the spur of the moment.

The components

To make the soup

- 1 tablespoon butter (unsalted)
- 1 leek, thoroughly washed and thinly sliced
- 1 big sliced sweet onion
- 212 pints chicken stock, unsalted
- 3 cups sweet peas, shelled
- 1 teaspoon of salt

To make the mint cream

- 12 cup yoghurt (plain)
- sour cream (12 cup)
- 1 tbsp. honey (ideally raspberry honey)

- 1 lemon's zest
- 1 lemon's juice
- 4 freshly minced mint leaves
- 12 mint leaves (for garnish)

Bee pollinated or produced foods are bolded.

Here's how it works:

1. Melt the butter in a 6-quart stockpot to create the soup. Cook, stirring occasionally, until the leek and onion are translucent, about 15 minutes.

2. Bring to a boil with the stock. Turn the heat to low and add the peas as soon as the liquid boils. 4 minutes of cooking (2 minutes if you use frozen peas). Remove the pan from the heat and set aside to cool. Season with salt.

3. Blend the soup in batches until completely smooth. You can also use a handheld immersion blender or a food processor, but a normal blender will provide the greatest consistency.

In a separate bowl, combine the yoghurt, sour cream, honey, lemon zest, and lemon juice to make the minted cream. Stir thoroughly. Minced mint is added last. Pulse until smooth with an immersion blender, a blender, or a food processor.

5. 5.Ladle the soup into bowls, top with 1 tablespoon of minted cream, then top with a fresh mint leaf. It's best served warm, not hot.

Honeyed Curry Dressing with Fresh Baby Vegetables

Serves 6

We've been making this dressing using maple syrup for years, which is great, especially if you're from Vermont like me. However, honey works nicely in this flexible and quick dipping sauce or salad dressing. It's worth a shot. If you have any sauce left over, spread it on a ham sandwich.

The components

To prepare the dressing

- Mayonnaise (12 cup)
- sour cream (12 cup)
- 2 tsp curry powder
- 2 tbsp. honey (ideally raspberry honey)

Regarding the vegetables

- 1–2 bunches baby carrots, sliced diagonally if necessary
- 1 bunch spring radishes, sliced diagonally if necessary
- 1 bunch baby turnips, sliced diagonally if necessary

Bee pollinated or produced foods are bolded.

Here's how it works:

1. In a small bowl, whisk together the mayonnaise, sour cream, curry powder, and honey to make the dressing. Warming the honey will make mixing easier (see below). Set aside for an hour or so in the refrigerator to allow the flavours to mingle.

2. 2.If the vegetables aren't fresh from the garden and aren't very small, they may need to be softly steamed. If so, cook the vegetables for 3 to 5 minutes, just until soft, in a steamer basket over boiling water. Turn off the heat and drain the liquid.

3. 3.In a large mixing bowl, combine the carrots, radishes, and turnips. Toss in the dressing to mix. Serve right away.

Honey That Warms

To make combining honey easier, soak the honey jar in warm water for a few minutes or run it under hot water.

Beets with Oranges and Blue Cheese from the Garden

As an appetiser, it serves 4 people.

Because pasture-raised cows eat a variety of grasses that rely on pollinators, blue cheese is boldfaced in the ingredients list. However, not all dairy cows are fed on pasture, so not all milk requires honeybees; however, bees pollinate a large number of grasses.

The components

- 1 bunch (approximately 1 pound) young beets with tops (the smaller the better)
- 1 navel orange, cut into quarters after peeling and removing white membranes
- Olive oil (extra virgin)
- Vinegar of red wine
- Sea salt
- black pepper, freshly ground
- 2 teaspoons blue cheese crumbles (I like Maytag)
- Dill leaves for garnish (optional)

Bee pollinated or produced foods are bolded.

Here's how it works:

1. Cut the greens from the beets as near to the beets as possible. If desired, save the greens for garnish.
2. 2.Steam the beets in a bamboo or stainless steel steamer until a fork easily pierces them, about 10 minutes. (Small beets cook rapidly, but larger ones take longer.) Fill a big dish halfway with cold water to create an ice bath.

3. 3.Plunge the beets into the ice bath after removing them from the steamer. The skins should be easy to remove (this is so much easier than peeling them).

4. Cut the beets into slices. On a large platter, arrange the beets and orange slices, drizzle with olive oil and vinegar, and season with salt and pepper to taste.

5. 5.Add the cheese just before serving. Garnish with the reserved beet greens or dill.

Raspberry Honey Glazed Seared Duck Breasts

Serves 2

If you don't want to roast a whole duck, seek for individual duck breasts in your grocery store's frozen food section. They cook fast and offer a delicious, elegant-looking but easy-to-prepare main entrée. I've also had terrific success slicing them and serving them as a passing hors d'oeuvre with a little raspberry jam.

The components

- 2 skin-on boneless duck breasts
- Salt, coarse
- black pepper, freshly ground
- 4 tbsp. honey (ideally raspberry honey)

- 12 cup raspberries, fresh

Bee pollinated or produced foods are bolded.

Here's how it works:

1. Use a very sharp knife to score the duck fat, being careful not to cut all the way through. Salt and pepper the duck breasts before serving.

2. 2.In a cast-iron skillet, fry the duck breasts skin side down for 5 minutes over high heat. Cook for another 5 to 7 minutes, or until the duck is cooked to your liking. (To check for doneness, use an instant-read thermometer — 125°F is unusual — or cut a small slit in the underside of the duck.) I love medium rare, so I cook it until it is pale pink in colour, about 130°F. After you remove it from the fire, it will continue to cook for a few minutes.) Place the duck on a warm serving plate.

2. 3.Reserve 2 tablespoons of the oil from the skillet. Return the skillet to the burner and add the saved duck grease over medium heat. Add the honey and 14 cup of raspberries to the mixture. Allow to thicken at a low temperature. If necessary, season with salt and pepper to taste.

4. 4.Just before serving, slice the duck breasts and arrange them on a tray or individual plates with the raspberry sauce on top. Serve with the remaining 14 cup raspberries as a garnish.

Baby Turnips Braised in Sugar

Serves 4

Spring is a particularly nice season for baby vegetables. Carrots, parsnips, turnips, and beets are readily available at our local farmers' markets in bunches of brand-new, bite-size root veggies. While I was never a fan of turnips as a child and despised them as an adolescent, now that I have access to these precious babies, I have a whole different perspective as an adult. We demonstrated how to make these, as well as applesauce and apple turnovers, to a class of first graders. This was without a doubt the group's favourite. The honey glaze complements the natural sweetness of the turnips in this recipe, making them a pleasure and a great addition to a light spring dinner.

The components

- 1 pound turnips, baby
- unsalted butter, 1–2 teaspoons
- a quarter cup of honey, preferably raspberry honey
- a quarter teaspoon of salt

Bee pollinated or produced foods are bolded.

Here's how it works:

1. If you have truly fresh baby turnips, simply take off the tops and root, leaving the turnip unpeeled. They'll be ready to cook

after a short rinsing. You may need to peel and cut the turnips into wedges if they aren't fresh from the ground. Maintain a large wedge size, roughly one full mouthful per chunk.

2. 2.In a cast-iron skillet, melt the butter over medium heat. Cook, stirring frequently, until the turnips can be pierced with a fork, 15 to 20 minutes. The turnips should have begun to brown, which is a positive sign.

Reduce the heat to a low setting. Continue to whisk while you drizzle the honey over the turnips. Cook for another 10 minutes or until the turnips caramelise and turn a chestnut colour.

4. Sprinkle with salt right before serving to balance and enhance the sweetness of the turnips. Enjoy!

Fresh Mint and Raspberry Granita

Serves 6

Granita is a straightforward dessert. Do not be frightened. You won't need any special equipment or devices; all you'll need is some fresh fruit, a little sugar, a freezer, and a few hours of your time. Take my word for it. I used fresh raspberries and raspberry honey as sweeteners for this variation.

The components

• 4 cups raspberries, fresh

- 13 cup honey, ideally raspberry honey, with additional honey if necessary
- 1 lemon's zest
- 1 teaspoon of lemon juice

6 sprigs fresh mint

Bee pollinated or produced foods are bolded.

Here's how it works:

1. In a medium bowl, place the raspberries. Over the berries, drizzle the honey, lemon zest, and lemon juice. Allow 15 minutes to sit.

2. Using a fork, mash the fruit mixture until fully combined but not puréed. Taste and, if desired, add additional honey.

3. 3.Pour the batter into a 9-inch square metal cake pan and freeze for 1 hour, covered. Remove from the freezer and break up any frozen clumps with a fork. Return to the freezer for another 2 hours or until hard. Remove the granita from the freezer and break it up into flakes with a fork in a chopping motion. Return to the freezer, covered. You can prepare this up to three days ahead of time.

4. 4. To serve, re-flake the granita and add a mint sprig to each serving.

The Robot

The drones are the colony's only male bees. The drone's sole purpose is to mate with a colony's virgin queen.

Unfortunately, the drone dies after mating with a queen, leaving the reproductive section of his body attached to his conquest. Drones don't do much else but forage, collect nectar and pollen, and assist with housekeeping and queen care.

When the active honey-making season ends and the temperature lowers, the workers, unwilling to maintain their non-productive brothers through the winter, throw them out of the hive and leave them to die in the cold. When the colony reactivates in the spring, the workers will allow freshly hatched drones to live, as they want to ensure that their colony's genetics are transferred to other hives.

Drones are distinguished by their size, which is smaller than that of the queen but larger than that of the workers. Their eyes, in particular, are significantly larger than those of worker bees.

Under an electron microscope, you can observe sight receptors mixed with scent receptors in a drone's eye, which allow the drones to identify a queen during her mating flights.

Fizzy Strawberry

This recipe makes enough preserves for eight drinks.

A gift of field-fresh berries, a table full of fresh fruit, and a friend informing me she had recently baked some strawberries in the oven inspired this chic nonalcoholic cocktail. I started by cooking my fruit in a sauté pan, and then everything else came into place.

The ginger ale from Blenheim is particularly powerful. You might prefer a conventional ginger ale like Canada Dry or Schweppes if you're serving children or those with less adventurous palates.

The components

To make the strawberry jam

• 1 cup stemmed strawberries

• 2 tbsp. honey (ideally raspberry honey)

For each drink,

• Depending on the size of your champagne flutes, 14–13 cup orange juice

• Depending on the size of your champagne flutes, 14–13 cup strong ginger ale (I like Blenheim)

• 1 lovely fresh strawberry

• 1 blood orange slice

• 3 raspberries (fresh)

Bee pollinated or produced foods are bolded.

Here's how it works:

1. In a small skillet, mix the strawberries and honey to make the preserves. Crush the berries and whisk the mixture with a wooden spoon until it is completely smooth. Cook for 5 minutes over medium heat, or until the consistency of jam. Allow time for cooling.

2. Pour 1 spoonful of preserves into the bottom of each champagne glass to make each cocktail. Fill the glass with orange juice. Fill the rest of the glass with ginger ale just before serving. Serve garnished with strawberry, blood orange, and raspberries.

Honey from Tulip Poplar

Color: A dark orange/amber colour.

Weak aroma; cooked fruits

Lightly sweet with a buttery finish and caramel notes

Aftertaste: A trace of toffee lingers on the tongue.

Tulip poplar honey is made from nectar collected from the blossoms of tulip poplar trees, which can be found throughout the eastern United States. Early in the spring, the fragrant flowers bloom, attracting bees and resulting in the first honey flows in many of these places.

In late April and early May, a large tulip poplar tree in my backyard blooms with flowers and bees. Considering how light the honey's flavour is, it's a surprise dark colour.

Brie with Strawberry Preserves in Puff Pastry

As an appetiser, it serves 20 people.

Brie is a delicious cheese on its own, but it's much better when paired with a little sweetness. A thin slice of Brie topped with a thin slice of fresh strawberry and a dab of sour cream or crème fraîche is a popular hors d'oeuvre at my café. This recipe takes those components and dresses them up a little. Any seasonal fruit can be used to make quick preserves. Make a quick jam if you have fruit that is getting too ripe.

The components

For the preservation of

- 2 pounds stemmed fresh strawberries
- 2 teaspoons honey, tulip poplar honey preferred
- 1 tbsp vanilla extract

For the wrapped cheese

- 1 frozen puff pastry sheet
- For the pastry, unbleached all-purpose flour
- 1 wheel of Brie cheese (about 2 pounds)

- 1 egg
- Serve with crackers or baguette pieces

Bee pollinated or produced foods are bolded.

Here's how it works:

1. Place the strawberries in a medium nonreactive saucepan over low heat to prepare the preserves. If you prefer chunky preserves, stir gently; if you prefer a smoother texture, stir vigorously. Cook until the berries are delicious and the texture is to your liking.

2. Stir in the honey until it is completely mixed. Cook, stirring occasionally, until the mixture thickens slightly, about 20 minutes. Mix in the vanilla extract. Note that you want a spreadable mixture. Stop cooking before you get to the fruit paste stage. Set aside the preserves.

3. Thaw the puff pastry according to the package instructions to produce the wrapped cheese. Depending on the type of pastry, this will take 30 to 45 minutes. It should be possible to unfold it without it breaking.

4. Preheat the oven to 475 degrees Fahrenheit.

5. 5.Stretch the pastry square on a lightly floured surface until it is about 14 inches long on each side. Place the pastry dough on top of a parchment-lined nonstick baking sheet.

6. 6.In the centre of the pastry square, place the cheese. 12 cup strawberry preserves, spooned on top of the cheese Stretch and draw two opposite corners of the pastry square over the edge of the cheese until the corners are about 4 inches above the centre of the cheese. With one hand, hold these corners.

7. 7.Bring the remaining two corners up to meet the first two corners, one at a time. Gather all of the corners and place them on top of the cheese. You can make creative forms with the ends, such as ribbons or leaves. Be inventive!

8. Whisk together the egg and 1 tablespoon of water. With a fork, thoroughly combine the ingredients. Using a pastry brush, apply the egg wash to the whole surface of the puff pastry. The baked pastry will be shinier and more appealing as a result.

9. Bake for 30 minutes, or until the puff pastry has risen and turned a toasted golden colour. If the cheese is particularly cold when you begin baking, it may take longer. Just keep an eye out for that golden hue.

Remove the pastry from the oven and set it aside to cool for 30 to 45 minutes before serving (unless you want a big pool of molten Brie running all over your serving table).

11. 11.Transfer the pastry to a serving tray using parchment paper (or one or two wide, flat spatulas). Throw away the parchment.

12. 12.Serve with crackers and brace yourself for a barrage of compliments from your guests.

What Happens When Bees Make Honey?

It's enough to make you shake your head in wonder at the process of manufacturing honey. How did they figure out everything?

Simply put, honey is manufactured from nectar collected by worker bees while foraging. Each excursion comprises visits to anywhere between 150 and 1,500 identical flowers. "Flower faithfulness" is the term for this. A bee collects a small amount of nectar from each flower visit and stores it in her "honey stomach," which is distinct from her "digestive stomach." A particular enzyme is added to the honey stomach's contents as she forages, converting the complex sugar in the nectar to the simple sugar found in honey. The nectar in her honey stomach can weigh almost as much as she does by the time she's ready to return to the hive, resulting in a low-altitude journey home.

When the bee returns to the hive, it regurgitates the enzyme-enhanced nectar one drop at a time into a waiting honeycomb cell. During the busiest times of the year, nectar is passed from a field bee to a house bee, who then transports it to the cell, freeing the field bee to embark on another foraging journey.

The nectar brought to the hive by field bees is roughly 80% water, which is far too watery. The hive's constant temperature of 95°F (35°C) begins to evaporate this water. By fanning the liquid with their wings, worker bees speed up the evaporation process until the nectar is roughly 17 percent water – the consistency humans know as honey. The workers next cover the filled cell in gorgeous, fresh white beeswax, which protects it from deterioration. It will remain in this state indefinitely. Honey discovered thousands of years ago in ancient Egyptian pyramids was still palatable.

Honey is produced by bees for their own nutritional needs and is stored for the winter. In my location, the rule of thumb is to make sure the bees have one full medium super of honey each hive, with at least 50 pounds of honey to get them through the winter. The beekeeper can harvest any additional honey.

Vichyssoise with new potatoes

Serves 6–8

Local new potatoes are available in the beginning of the summer if you live in a latitude comparable to mine (the middle of the country). If you don't have access to them or can't find them, look for the best, smallest potatoes you can find. Yukon Golds are my favourite because they add a wonderful pop of colour to this soup, which is a great way to start an early summer dinner on the porch. Are you having lunch with the ladies? Serve this to them!

The components

12 cup unsalted butter (1 stick)

- 6 well-washed leeks, sliced into 12-inch slices
- 12 cup (1 small sweet onion, chopped into medium cubes)
- 6 cups chicken or vegetable stock, unsalted
- 312 cup young potatoes, diced (skin on)
- Salt
- black pepper, freshly ground
- 1 gallon whole milk
- 2 cups sour cream
- 1 quart thick cream (optional)
- Garnish with watercress sprigs

Bee pollinated or produced foods are bolded.

Here's how it works:

1. In a large soup pot over medium heat, melt the butter. Sauté the leeks and onion for 5 to 7 minutes, or until transparent. Allowing them to brown is not a good idea. Add the potatoes

and stock to the pot. Reduce the heat to low and cook for 25 minutes, or until the potatoes are tender.

2. 2.Using an immersion blender, pulse the liquid until it is as smooth as you desire. It's best to stop before it's totally puréed, as some texture is beneficial.

3. Taste and season with salt and pepper (the amounts will vary depending on the saltiness of your stock). Stir in the milk and half-and-half until thoroughly combined. Cook for 15 minutes over low heat, taking care not to allow the soup boil. Allow to cool after removing from the heat. Refrigerate until completely chilled.

4. 4.Ladle the mixture into individual dishes or cups. If desired, drizzle each bowl with 1 tablespoon heavy cream and a sprig or two of fresh watercress.

Salad with strawberries and honeyed balsamic vinegar reduction

Serves 4

If you have leftover balsamic vinegar reduction, use it to make a refreshing and refined dessert: a bowl of fresh strawberries with the reduction.

The components

Reduced balsamic vinegar

- 1 tablespoon balsamic vinegar
- 14 cup honey, tulip poplar honey preferred

To make the salad

- 1 pound spring mix greens
- 2 cups half-sliced fresh strawberries
- Extra-virgin olive oil (13 cup)
- 12 cup feta cheese, crumbled
- 12 cup toasted slivered almonds (optional)

Bee pollinated or produced foods are bolded.

Here's how it works:

1. Place the balsamic vinegar in a small nonreactive pot to prepare the balsamic reduction. Bring to a boil, then turn down to a low heat. Cook for around 15 minutes, or until the volume has been decreased by half.

2. 2.Add the honey and heat until the mixture thickens to the consistency of a thick syrup that coats the back of a spoon easily. (At the end of the cooking process, watch carefully since it can easily get too thick, in which case you may need to dilute it with a little water.) You're hoping for a honey-like consistency. Turn off the heat.

3. Arrange the mixed greens on a serving plate to make the salad. On top of the greens, scatter the strawberries.

4. Sprinkle the salad with olive oil just before serving, then drizzle a thin stream of balsamic reduction over the top, making sure to get it on the berries. Sprinkle the cheese and sliced almonds on top, if using.

Smoky Onion Crust on Wild Salmon

Serves 5–6

My friend Sally is from a little island in the Pacific Northwest, where she grew up roasting salmon on wood planks on the beach. She told me about her father's recipe, which included a special herb mixture. I made my own, despite never having tried his. No beach? Don't be concerned. My variation is prepared in your backyard over a smoky charcoal fire.

While the salmon is delightful hot, the flavours enhance with time, making this an excellent leftover or the foundation for a delicious chunky smoked-salmon salad.

The components

• 1 cup grilling chips (hardwood) (Hickory, Maple, and Alderwood are good options)

12 cup unsalted butter (1 stick)

• 1 tablespoon salt from Johnny's (see sidebar on following page)

• 2 teaspoons honey, tulip poplar honey preferred

• 4 sliced medium sweet onions (such as Vidalia or Walla Walla)

• 1 side skin-on wild Alaskan salmon (about 3 pounds)

Bee pollinated or produced foods are bolded.

Here's how it works:

1. Light a charcoal fire in your grill about 112 hours before you plan to eat. Allow the coals to cool to a medium temperature before starting to cook. Alternatively, if using a gas grill, start a medium heat when ready to cook. While the onions are cooking, soak a handful of wood chips in water.

2. 2.In a large skillet, melt the butter over low heat. Season with seasoned salt, honey, and onions (you'll have a large pile of onions, but they'll soften and shrink as they cook). Cook, stirring occasionally, for 45 minutes or until the onions are very fully cooked and resemble a thick mash, almost like paste.

3. Place the fish on the grill, skin side down. To protect it from adhering to the grill, place it on a piece of aluminium foil (taking cautious not to cover the entire grill surface with foil), but if your grill is properly seasoned, you can skip this step. On top of the salmon, spread the onion mixture. Close the grill cover and cook for 15 minutes on low heat.

4. 4.Insert the moistened wood chips into the coals after opening the cover. This will result in a hazy flame. Close the grill lid and smoke the salmon for another 15 minutes or more, depending on the thickness of the fish. To see if the fish is alive, gently probe it with your finger. I want my fish slightly underdone, so I remove it off the grill when it is still soft. Continue to cook until the meat is firmer if you prefer your fish well done.

5. Place the fish on a serving platter and cover loosely with foil. Allow for 5 to 10 minutes before serving.

salt for seasoning

If you can't find Johnny's Seasoning Salt, combine the following ingredients to produce a suitable substitute: 1 teaspoon granulated garlic, 1 teaspoon granulated sugar, 14 teaspoon paprika, 1 teaspoon freshly ground black pepper

Tulip Poplar Honey–Mustard Vinaigrette with Haricots Verts

Serves 8–10

Here's how to keep vegetables looking bright and fresh when cooking. You may make them ahead of time if you want, which is very useful on a hot June night.

The vinaigrette, too, can be made ahead of time. This recipe makes more vegetables than you'll need, but it's so wonderful that you can save the leftovers for tomorrow. It's far superior to those bottled concoctions. If you can't obtain tulip poplar honey, find a local beekeeper and collect from his or her early honey flow - something light will suffice.

The components

- red wine vinegar (3 teaspoons)
- 1 tablespoon honey (tulip poplar preferred)
- 1 tablespoon Dijon mustard, coarsely ground
- 1 cup high-quality extra-virgin olive oil
- Sea salt
- black pepper, freshly ground
- 2 pounds haricots verts, fresh (baby French green beans)

Bee pollinated or produced foods are bolded.

Here's how it works:

1. In a medium mixing basin, whisk together the vinegar, honey, and mustard. Drizzle the oil in a thin stream into the mixing bowl, whisking constantly until fully combined. This will emulsify the mixture, allowing it to stay combined. If required, season with salt and pepper. Keep it aside until you're ready to utilise it.

2. Bring a big pot of water to a rolling boil. Fill a large mixing basin halfway with ice water. Plunge the green beans into the

boiling water while keeping an eye on them. The beans will become a bright green colour after about 1 minute (the timing will vary based on the age of the beans). Remove them from the pot immediately and submerge them in ice water to stop the cooking and keep them brilliant green. Remove them from the ice water once they've cooled and drain them in a colander.

3. Arrange the beans on a plate to serve. Serve the beans with the vinaigrette drizzled on top.

Crème de Fromage

Serves 4

This is my take on one of my mother's favourite dishes. This is a classic dessert that, like so many others of its kind, is excellent. You'll need one of those 15-ounce porcelain moulds with little holes, usually heart-shaped, as well as cheesecloth to line the mould. Aside from that, this is a straightforward dish. Yes, it is filling, but modest portions can be served. Moderation in all things permits you to indulge in minor pleasures now and then, right?

The components

- 8 oz. cream cheese
- whipping cream (34 cup)
- Grand Marnier (2 teaspoons)

• 2 tablespoons honey (tulip poplar honey preferred), plus more for sprinkling (optional)

• Garnish with fresh strawberries

Bee pollinated or produced foods are bolded.

Here's how it works:

1. In a large mixing bowl, beat the cream cheese and half of the cream until extremely frothy. 1 tablespoon honey and 1 tablespoon Grand Marnier 1 minute more whipping

2. 2.In a separate dish, whip the remaining cream with the remaining 1 tablespoon honey until firm. Make care to pause before making butter!

Fold the whipped cream into the cheese mixture in thirds.

4. Pour the combined cheese and whipped cream mixture into a 15-ounce mould lined with cheesecloth. Refrigerate for at least three hours or overnight.

Unmold onto a serving dish when ready to serve. Serve with strawberries and a drizzle of honey, if desired.

Spritzers with Rosemary and Melon

Serves 8

Make this drink using the ripest, most aromatic melon you can find, especially if you're hosting a swanky sitting brunch. Begin or end with this. In either case, you'll get a lot of compliments and requests for the recipe.

The components

- 1 seeded cantaloupe, scooped into balls using a melon scoop
- 8 teaspoons honey, tulip poplar honey preferred
- 8 rosemary sprigs, fresh
- Sparkling wine that is sweet (or Champagne)
- Garnish with fresh raspberries

Bee pollinated or produced foods are bolded.

Here's how it works:

1. Put 5 melon balls in each of the 8 martini glasses around 30 minutes before your guests arrive. Drizzle 1 teaspoon honey into each glass and garnish with a sprig of rosemary pierced into a melon ball. Allow time to pass.

2. Fill each glass with sparkling wine when ready to serve. Serve with raspberries as a garnish. The rosemary aroma will mingle with the melon and honey as the visitors drink. If desired, serve the melon balls with a fancy fork or small spoon.

CPSIA information can be obtained
at www.ICGtesting.com
Printed in the USA
LVHW060215160722
723616LV00015B/792

9 781804 768457